Home-Cooked Cancer Diet for Dogs

Easy, Nutrient-Packed Recipes

Noel M. Reeder

Table of Contents

Chapter I:Introduction

In dogs, cancer can be prevented and treated in large part by eating a balanced diet. Research has repeatedly demonstrated that a healthy, well-balanced diet has a major influence on a dog's general health and wellness, including how likely they are to contract certain diseases like cancer. A nutritious diet is crucial for managing and preventing cancer in dogs for the following reasons:

Promotes Immune System Function: To identify and eradicate aberrant cells before they develop into tumors, the immune system must be powerful and resilient. The immune system can detect and eliminate precancerous cells with more efficiency when it receives the nutrients it needs from a balanced diet.

Diminishes Inflammation: Prolonged inflammation has been associated with a higher risk of several cancer kinds. Inflammation can be decreased and the risk of cancer can be decreased with a nutritious diet rich in anti-inflammatory foods such as whole grains, fruits, and vegetables high in antioxidants, and omega-3 fatty acids.

Encourages Weight Management: Excess body fat raises the synthesis of hormones and growth factors that aid in the development of cancer, making obesity a major risk factor for cancer in dogs. A balanced diet and frequent exercise can help maintain a healthy weight and lower the risk of malignancies linked to obesity.

Improves Treatment Outcomes: If a dog gets cancer, conventional cancer therapies like radiation, chemotherapy, and surgery will work better when the dog eats a nutritious diet. Antioxidants and omega-3 fatty acids are two examples of foods that might lessen the harmful effects of radiation and chemotherapy while safeguarding healthy cells and tissues.

Lastly, nutritious food may significantly enhance a dog's quality of life both before and after cancer treatment. To keep the dog comfortable and have a high quality of life throughout the illness and its treatments, a proper diet can help reduce symptoms like nausea, vomiting, and appetite loss.

Choosing healthful, natural foods that offer the nutrients required to boost a dog's immune system, lower inflammation, control weight, increase the efficacy of therapy, and enhance overall quality of life is a summary of home-cooked cancer diet alternatives for dogs. The following broad principles can be applied when creating a homemade cancer diet for dogs:

High-quality proteins: Protein is necessary for tissue growth and repair, muscle maintenance, and immune system support. Lean meat, chicken, fish, and eggs are good sources of protein. If at all feasible, seek out organic, grass-fed, wild-caught, and pasture-raised types;

they tend to be fewer toxins and richer in nutrients than their conventionally reared counterparts.

Anti-Inflammatory components: Reducing chronic inflammation and lowering the risk of cancer can be achieved by including anti-inflammatory components such as omega-3 fatty acids, antioxidants, and phytochemicals. Examples include bright fruits and vegetables like berries, tomatoes, bell peppers, and leafy greens; nuts and seeds like walnuts, flaxseeds, and chia seeds; coldwater fish like salmon, sardines, and mackerel; and spices like turmeric, cinnamon, and ginger.

Whole Grains: Whole grains are great providers of fiber, complex carbs, and important vitamins and minerals. Examples of such foods are brown rice, quinoa, millet, and buckwheat. They should, however, be well prepared and consumed in moderation since overindulging in them might result in weight gain and other health problems.

Healthy Fats: You may boost the quality of your skin and coat, provide your energy, and help your body absorb fat-soluble vitamins by including moderate amounts of healthy fats like avocado, coconut oil, olive oil, nuts, and seeds. Steer clear of bad fats like shortening, margarine, and hydrogenated oils since these can worsen inflammation and cause heart disease.

Reduced Processed Ingredients: It's usually advised to limit processed and packaged meals since they frequently include preservatives, additives, and other chemicals that can be harmful to a dog's health. Fresh, whole foods that are cooked simply and without needless processing are preferable.

Customization: Depending on factors including age, breed, size, exercise level, and present health, every dog has different nutritional demands. For this reason, it's critical to collaborate with a veterinarian or canine nutritionist to create a customized home-cooked cancer diet that accounts for each of these variables.

Harmony and Diversification: It's crucial to feed a range of foods and strive for balance between macronutrients (protein, carbs, and fats) and micronutrients (vitamins and minerals) to make sure a dog gets all the nutrients they need.

Rotation: Changing meal plans and ingredients regularly lowers the chance of boredom or pickiness in dogs and helps prevent deficiencies in any one nutrient.

Safety Measures: Food safety requires that all meats, poultry, and fish be cooked completely to eradicate any germs or parasites. Additionally, make sure to store leftovers right away, toss uneaten food after a few days, and chill all food fully before serving.

Pet owners may prepare tasty, nourishing, and efficient home-cooked cancer foods that support their dog's health and welfare both before and after cancer treatment by following these principles and receiving expert advice as needed.

Chapter II: Understanding Canine Nutritional Needs of Cancer

The Role of Nutrition in Cancer Prevention and Treatment

The role that nutrition plays in both preventing and treating cancer in dogs cannot be overstated, since their ability to fend off the disease and recover from it may be significantly impacted by their food. A dog's capacity to prevent and treat cancer may be impacted by their food in the following ways:

- Increasing Immune Function: A strong immune system is necessary to identify and get rid of abnormal cells before they turn into cancer. Nutrition is crucial for preserving immune function because some nutrients, like vitamin C, vitamin E, zinc, selenium, and beta-carotene, operate as strong antioxidants that help protect cells from damage caused by free radicals.

- Controlling Cell Growth and Division: Nutrients involved in DNA synthesis and regulation, such as folate, vitamin B12, and methionine, are essential in controlling cell growth and division. Deficits in several nutrients have been linked to an increased risk of cancer.

- Modulating Inflammation: Chronic inflammation has been discovered to have an impact on a variety of cancer kinds. Consuming anti-inflammatory foods can help reduce inflammation and reduce the risk of cancer. Examples of these foods include curcumin, resveratrol, quercetin, and omega-3 fatty acids.

- Managing Body Weight: Excess body fat causes the production of pro-inflammatory cytokines and adipokines, which encourage tumor formation and angiogenesis. This has been linked to an increased risk of cancer in dogs. Eating a balanced diet and exercising frequently to maintain a healthy weight helps reduce the risk of cancer.

- Detoxification: Toxins from food, water, air, and the environment can accumulate in the body and cause cancer. Glutathione, sulforaphane, and indoles are among the substances found in cruciferous vegetables that can support the body's detoxification efforts and help in the elimination of harmful contaminants.

- Modifying Gene Expression: Recent research indicates that several nutrients, including lycopene from tomatoes, genistein from soybeans, and epigallocatechin gallate (EGCG) from green tea, might alter the patterns of gene expression in cancer cells, hence inhibiting the growth and metastasis of the cells.

- Increasing Energy: A dog's energy reserves may be depleted by cancer treatment such as chemotherapy and radiation therapy, leaving them listless. Serving a nutrient-dense, easily digested meal can help boost energy and speed up the healing process.

- Reduction of Side Effects: Radiation and chemotherapy can induce painful side effects such as nausea, vomiting, and appetite loss. Giving dogs on medication tasty, easily digested, and stomach-friendly food can help alleviate these symptoms and improve their quality of life.

- Boosting General Health: A dog that eats a well-rounded, species-appropriate diet will be healthier all around, which will help them resist cancer and its treatments. Better digestion, boosted immunity, less inflammation, stronger teeth, bones, muscles, joints, and organs, as well as more stable emotions and behavior, are all part of this.

It's important to keep in mind that although food cannot prevent cancer, it can improve the results of traditional cancer therapies. The optimal diet plan for a dog's specific kind and stage of cancer should be determined by consulting with a veterinarian or canine nutritionist, as each dog's cancer case is unique and needs individualized attention and care.

Nutrients that are beneficial for dogs with Cancer

Whole-Grain Protein

Protein is a vital nutrient for dogs with cancer because it promotes immunity, helps with wound healing, tissue regeneration, maintenance, and repair, and keeps muscle mass during stressful or sick periods. When dogs get cancer therapy, they may become weak and have muscle wasting due to malnourishment, decreased appetite, cachexia, or direct muscle tissue damage from the disease. As a result, increasing protein intake is even more crucial to preserving the dog's physical condition and muscular composition.

For dogs with cancer, protein has the following benefits:
- Preserve Muscular Mass: Eating adequate protein can help stop the debility and loss of muscular mass that are caused by cancer and its treatments.

Protein-rich diets have been demonstrated to improve nitrogen retention, which is essential for maintaining strength and muscle mass.

- Boosts Immunity: Protein-based amino acids like arginine, histidine, and glutamine are important for immune system function and help produce antibodies, white blood cells, and other immune components.

- Protein is necessary for the repair of damaged tissues and for promoting rapid wound healing after surgery or other trauma. Increasing your protein consumption helps minimize issues and speed up the healing process.

- Provides Energy: Although fats and carbohydrates are often the primary energy sources, protein may also be utilized as a fallback when needed. This is particularly beneficial for cancer-stricken dogs or those receiving cancer treatments that interfere with their ability to consume or absorb other macronutrients.

- Contributes to Drug Metabolism: Many cancer-treating drugs are metabolized by enzymes, which produce amino acids from protein. Adequate protein ensures optimal drug metabolism and excretion, reducing the risk of toxic buildup or unwanted reactions.

- When picking protein sources for dogs with cancer, look for high-quality, easily digestible options such as lean meats, poultry, fish, eggs, and dairy products. Organic, grass-fed, wild-caught, and pasture-grown varieties frequently have higher nutritional content and lower pollution levels than their conventionally farmed equivalents. Furthermore, boiling, poaching, steaming, and roasting are examples of culinary techniques that further break down protein structures, increasing their absorbability and digestibility.

However, excessive protein consumption can further strain the kidneys and liver and lead to organ failure or dysfunction, therefore it's important to properly monitor intake. It is highly recommended that you seek veterinarian supervision to establish the proper quantity and frequency of protein supplements, considering the unique needs and overall health of the dog.

Omega-3 fatty acids

The potential medicinal applications of polyunsaturated fats, sometimes referred to as omega-3 fatty acids, in the treatment and prevention of cancer in people and animals have generated a great deal of attention. Eicosapentaenoic acid (EPA) and docosahexaenoic acid (DHA), the two main forms of omega-3 fatty acids, have demonstrated anti-inflammatory, antiangiogenic, antimetastatic, and apoptotic properties that may be helpful for cancer-stricken dogs.

Some benefits of omega-3 fatty acids for dogs with cancer include the following:

- Diminish Inflammation: Owing to their potent anti-inflammatory properties, omega-3 fatty acids have the potential to mitigate chronic inflammation resulting from cancer and its treatment. By competing with arachidonic acid, another fatty acid involved in the synthesis of pro-inflammatory prostaglandins and leukotrienes, they suppress the inflammatory response.

- Stop Angiogenesis: Tumors require the development of new blood vessels to receive oxygen and nourishment as they grow. Angiogenesis is the term for this process. Omega-3 fatty acids have been shown to inhibit angiogenesis, which limits the availability of oxygen and nutrients to cancer cells and delays the development of tumors.

- Start Apoptosis: Apoptosis, also referred to as programmed cell death, is a normal physiological process that eliminates unhealthy or undesirable cells. Research has demonstrated that apoptosis, a process that helps eliminate cancer cells and prevents them from proliferating, may be triggered by omega-3 fatty acids.

- Enhance Cachexia: Cachexia is a severe form of muscle atrophy marked by weakness, a gradual loss of body weight, and a worse quality of life. It has been shown that omega-3 fatty acids improve cachectic conditions by increasing appetite, promoting fat storage, and maintaining muscle mass.

- Boost Response to Therapy: It has been suggested that omega-3 fatty acids might enhance the efficacy of some cancer therapies by blocking resistance mechanisms and raising responsiveness to chemotherapeutic medicines. Additionally, they may lessen the negative side effects of cancer treatment, such as neuropathy, myopathy, and cardiotoxicity.

- Dogs can benefit greatly from eating cold-water fish, including herring, sardines, anchovies, mackerel, and salmon. Plant-based sources of alpha-linolenic acid (ALA), which is a precursor to EPA and DHA, include flaxseed, chia seed, and hemp seed. However, dogs do not convert ALA very well. You may wish to take fish oil supplements that have been molecularly distilled to remove contaminants like mercury, dioxins, and PCBs to maximize the absorption of omega-3 fatty acids.

As with any dietary intervention, consult a veterinarian or canine nutritionist before introducing omega-3 fatty acids into a dog's daily diet. The right dosage and frequency must be determined after taking the dog's particular needs and health into account. When used improperly, it might have unfavorable side effects including weakened immune system function, slower wound healing, or bleeding issues. For cancer-stricken dogs, it is imperative to regularly monitor and consult with a healthcare professional to ensure the safe and effective use of omega-3 fatty acids.

Antioxidants

Antioxidants are compounds that protect cells from the oxidative damage caused by free radicals, which are unstable molecules generated by environmental exposure or metabolic processes. Free radicals may react with biological membranes, proteins, lipids, and DNA to cause irreparable damage as well as inflammation, aging, and disease. Antioxidants scavenge free radicals, neutralizing them and safeguarding the integrity and functionality of cells.

Dogs with cancer can benefit from antioxidants in several ways, such as:

- Combat Oxidative Stress: The increased generation of free radicals by cancer cells generates oxidative stress, which deteriorates adjacent healthy tissues and reduces immune system effectiveness. Antioxidants counteract these free radicals, reestablishing redox balance and assisting the immune system in mounting an effective attack against cancer cells.

- Boost Immune Surveillance: A healthy immune system depends on efficient surveillance mechanisms that can recognize and eliminate alterations in cells at an early stage of development. Antioxidants enhance immunological surveillance by shielding immune cells from oxidative damage and preserving their structural integrity and functional capacity.

- Boost Chemotherapy Efficiency: According to research, including antioxidants in chemotherapy may make the medications more cytotoxic to cancer cells while protecting healthy cells from inadvertent damage.

- Reduce Adverse Reactions: Antioxidants may reduce the severity of side effects such as thrombocytopenia, oral mucositis, nausea, vomiting, and neutropenia by preventing the generation of free radicals caused by chemotherapy.

- Reduced Inflammation and Oxidative Stress: Antioxidants have demonstrated potential in mitigating angiogenesis, reducing the danger of metastases, and delaying the progression of cancer.

- Dog cancer diets often include antioxidants like polyphenols, flavonoids, and carotenoids, as well as vitamins C, E, and A, which are found in fruits, vegetables, and herbs. For instance, vitamin E has radioprotective and neuroprotective qualities, while vitamin C can boost immunity and cooperate with chemotherapy medications. Polyphenols and flavonoids, which are abundant in plant-derived ingredients including green tea, pine bark, and grape seed extract, exhibit exceptional antioxidant qualities and help fortify immunological responses.

While antioxidants offer many advantages, they can also have disadvantages. For instance, many chemotherapy medications may become less effective when used in large quantities of antioxidants. Moreover, combining various antioxidants may have paradoxical effects, so it's important to choose and titrate them carefully depending on the demands of your dog. It is crucial to initially consult a veterinarian or canine nutritionist to decide the proper antioxidant selections, dosages, and delivery schedules based on the specific conditions and cancer diagnosis of the dog. Regular reassessments and modifications may be required to consider evolving clinical conditions.

Fiber

Any dog's cancer diet should include a lot of fiber because it has so many health advantages. Among these advantages are:

- Control of Gut Motility: Fiber facilitates regular bowel movements and prevents constipation, which can occasionally result from cancer treatment. It also helps fecal material pass through the gastrointestinal tract.

- Microbiota Modulation: In the colon, soluble fibers ferment fast and form short-chain fatty acids (SCFAs), which boost the growth of good gut microbes and, as a consequence, improve the gut barrier and inhibit bacterial translocation.

- Controlled Appetite: Eating meals high in fiber makes you feel full, which helps you avoid overindulging and lose weight. Given the increased risk of cancer associated with fat, this is particularly crucial for dogs who are prone to obesity.

- Blood sugar regulation: Fiber helps delay stomach emptying and hinders the absorption of carbs, resulting in more regular postprandial glucose fluctuations and less insulin being produced. Such consequences become noteworthy given the correlation between hyperglycemia and worse cancer prognosis.

Xenobiotic Clearance: By accelerating transit times and binding harmful molecules, insoluble fibers lessen the quantity of mutagenic or carcinogenic substances absorbed via the digestive system.

- Psyllium husk, pumpkin puree, ground flaxseed, and nutrient-dense grains like brown rice or quinoa are occasionally included in dog cancer diets as fiber sources. However, caution must be used when it comes to the amount and kind of fiber consumed, as an excess may result in cramps, diarrhea, bloating, or gas, which might adversely affect the absorption of nutrients and patient comfort. Since everyone has a different tolerance, it is vital to increase the amount of fiber gradually while monitoring closely. Working with a veterinarian or dog nutritionist enables the purposeful addition of fiber components according to the specific requirements and cancer profile of the dog.

Foods to avoid

Given the influence that poor feeding habits may have on the progression of the disease, the efficacy of therapy, and the overall health of the dog, it is essential to know which foods are best avoided by dogs diagnosed with cancer. Several dietary groups should be avoided, primarily:

- Processed meats and sausages: According to many studies, there is a higher risk of colorectal cancer in people who consume processed meats, which include preservatives such as sodium nitrite and nitrate. Similar mammalian mechanisms imply that our canine companions most likely experience similar outcomes. As a result, processed meats of any kind should never be served to dogs suffering from cancer.

- Artificial Sweeteners: Xylitol is one of the most harmful artificial sweeteners for dogs. They may result in hypoglycemia, convulsions, and potentially fatal liver damage. It is advised that dogs receiving cancer therapy stay away from artificial sweeteners entirely, even though there is no conclusive evidence linking them to the disease.

- Refined Carbohydrates: Simple sugars have no nutritional value at all and lead to abrupt increases and decreases in blood sugar levels, which worsen inflammation and insulin resistance throughout the body. Rather, choose whole grain substitutes that include slowly digesting complex carbohydrates that promote prolonged energy release and elevated glycemic stability.

- Hydrogenated Oils: It is commonly recognized that the trans fats included in partly hydrogenated oils induce endothelial dysfunction and vascular inflammation, which can worsen the development and metastasis of cancer. Select exclusively unsaturated oils, with a preference for mono- and polyunsaturated sources including flaxseed, sesame, and extra virgin olive oil.

- Genetically Modified Crops: The research indicates that genetically modified crops may be linked to the onset of cancer, but it is still in its early stages. Until proven otherwise, it appears reasonable to use non-GMO veggies when designing cancer-preventive dog meals.

- Foods Contaminated by Mycotoxins: Mold infestations can create mycotoxins, which are chemical compounds that have the potential to inhibit the immune system, cause cancer, and have estrogenic effects on food. Food products should be thoroughly inspected for signs of degradation; perishables should be eaten right away to stop fungus development, and refrigeration is recommended for storage.

Refusing to include these food groups promotes safer, more effective dog cancer diets, which improves health outcomes. On the other hand, consulting with veterinarians or dog nutritionists guarantees thorough, personalized advice that is by unique canine traits and cancer profiles.

Chapter III. Easy and Nutritious Homemade Recipes for Dogs with Cancer

Breakfast recipes

Turkey and vegetable omelet
Servings: 2-3 servings

Prep Time: 10 minutes

Cook Time: 15 minutes

Total Time: 25 minutes

Description: Start your dog's day with a protein-packed, nutrient-dense turkey and vegetable omelette, brimming with cancer-fighting ingredients!

Ingredients:
3 large eggs, preferably organic and cage-free
¼ cup unsweetened almond milk or goat's milk
½ teaspoon dried basil
½ teaspoon dried oregano
Freshly ground black pepper, to taste
¾ cup chopped cooked turkey breast, no skin or bone

⅓ cup sautéed mixed vegetables (bell peppers, mushrooms, spinach, etc.)
1 tablespoon extra virgin olive oil
Optional: A sprinkle of nutritional yeast for added B vitamins

Instructions:
- Crack open the eggs into a mixing bowl, pour in the almond milk or goat's milk, then whisk until yolk and whites combine uniformly.
- Sprinkle basil, oregano, and black pepper into the egg mixture, blending well.
- Heat olive oil in a medium skillet over medium heat. Once warm, introduce the chopped turkey breast and cook for approximately 2 minutes, just long enough to reheat the meat.
- Pour the beaten eggs over the heated turkey, distributing evenly. Allow the edges to set slightly, around 1 minute.
- Scatter the sautéed veggie blend onto one half of the partially cooked omelet, then fold the remaining half gently over the filling.
- Lower heat to medium-low and cover the skillet, letting the omelet complete cooking for about 5-7 minutes, or until fully set.
- Remove from heat and transfer to a plate, slicing into bite-sized pieces once cooled sufficiently.

Optionally, dust with nutritional yeast for an extra dose of B vitamins.

- Serve immediately, reserving any leftovers covered in the fridge for up to three days. Enjoy!

Quinoa porridge with berries

Servings: 2-3 servings

Prep Time: 5 minutes

Cook Time: 20 minutes

Total Time: 25 minutes

Description: Deliver a warming, energizing start to your dog's morning routine with this delightfully simple yet packed full of goodness – Quinoa Porridge with Berries!

Ingredients:

½ cup organic quinoa, rinsed and drained

1 cup filtered water

½ cup unsweetened almond milk or goat's milk

1 small ripe banana, mashed

½ teaspoon ground cinnamon

⅛ teaspoon sea salt

1 teaspoon raw honey or maple syrup (optional)

½ cup frozen mixed berries (blueberries, strawberries, cherries, raspberries)
Optional toppings: shredded coconut, crushed almonds, chia seeds

Instructions:
Combine quinoa and water in a saucepan, bringing it to a boil. Then, lower the heat, cover, and let simmer for roughly 15 minutes or until tender and the liquid has been absorbed.

Mix in almond milk or goat's milk, mashed banana, cinnamon, and salt, heating everything together for a couple of minutes. You may wish to incorporate an optional sweetener here too. Ensure the temperature isn't piping hot for your pup, though.

Take the pan off the stove and throw in frozen berries, giving them a moment to soften amidst the warmth of the cereal mix. Feel free to reserve a few for a pretty presentation later.

Spoon out enticing portions into your dog's dish, scattering chosen toppings generously for bonus texture and flavors. Keep leftovers sealed in the fridge for up to three days.

Remember - always double-check with your vet or canine nutrition specialist regarding portion sizes and ingredient compatibility in line with your doggo's bespoke needs and cancer journey. Happy noshing!

Lunch recipes

Chicken and sweet potato stew

Servings: 4-6 servings

Prep Time: 15 minutes

Cook Time: 30 minutes

Total Time: 45 minutes

Description: Pamper your deserving dog with this irresistibly savory and comforting chicken and sweet potato stew bursting with vibrant veggies and medicinal herbs!

Ingredients:

1 lb boneless, skinless organic chicken breasts or thighs, cut into chunks
2 tbsp olive oil or coconut oil
1 medium yellow onion, finely chopped
3 cloves garlic, minced
2 cups low-sodium organic chicken stock

1 medium sweet potato, peeled and cubed
1 cup chopped green beans
1 cup chopped carrots
1 cup peas (fresh or frozen)
1 bay leaf
1 sprig rosemary
1 sprig thyme
Salt and pepper to taste

Instructions:
Begin by heating oil in a Dutch oven or deep skillet over medium heat. Introduce the chicken pieces and cook until lightly golden, turning occasionally. Transfer cooked chicken to a clean plate.

Within the same pan, sweat onions and garlic until fragrant and translucent. Return the seared chicken to the pot alongside chicken stock, sweet potatoes, green beans, carrots, peas, and seasonings.

Bring the contents to a simmer, placing a lid on top whilst keeping it slightly ajar. Let it bubble away for around 20-25 minutes, granting ample opportunity for the flavors to meld harmoniously.

Check the doneness of veggies, removing the stew from heat once they reach the desired consistency. Discard herb stalks before doling out sumptuous portions into your eagerly waiting companion's bowl. Any residual stew can safely remain refrigerated for up to four days.

As ever, never neglect to verify portion sizes and ingredient appropriateness with your trusted vet or canine nutrition aficionado, accounting for your darling buddy's exclusive health concerns and restrictions. Bon appétit!

Fish and brown rice casserole
Servings: 4-6 servings

Prep Time: 15 minutes

Cook Time: 45 minutes

Total Time: 1 hour

Description: Lavish your treasured friend with this tantalizingly tempting and nurturing fish and brown rice casserole, teeming with precious omega-3 fatty acids and valuable vitamins!

Ingredients:
1 lb wild-caught cod filets, skin removed and cut into chunks
1 cup organic brown rice, rinsed
2 cups water or low-sodium organic vegetable broth

1 medium yellow onion, finely chopped
2 cloves garlic, minced
1 cup chopped broccoli florets
1 cup chopped summer squash
1 cup halved cherry tomatoes
1 tbsp olive oil or coconut oil
Juice of 1 lemon
Zest of 1 lemon
1 tbsp chopped parsley
1 tbsp chopped dill
Salt and pepper to taste

Instructions:
Initiate by heating oil in a large oven-safe skillet or Dutch oven over medium heat. Integrate onions and garlic, sautéing until aromatic and glassy.

Amalgamate rice, water or broth, broccoli, squash, tomatoes, lemon juice, zest, herbs, and seasonings within the pan. Simmer for 10 minutes, permitting liquids to encircle the ingredients lovingly.

Place fish delicately atop the medley, dispersing it equitably amongst the diverse elements. Slide the pan into a preheated oven, setting it to 375°F (190°C) for approximately 30-35 minutes, or until the fish effortlessly flakes apart and the rice achieves perfect tenderness.

Retrieve the captivating creation from the fiery embrace of the oven, embellishing it with a final shower of herbs if preferred. Present the divine dish proudly before your fortunate recipient, secure in the knowledge that leftovers will retain freshness for up to five days tucked snugly away inside the refrigerator.

Of course, bear in mind the necessity of confirming portion sizes and ingredient aptitude with your esteemed veterinarian or canine nutrition guardian angel, cognisant of your marvelous companion's special health requisitions and limitations.

Beef and broccoli stir fry
Servings: 4-6 servings

Prep Time: 15 minutes

Cook Time: 15 minutes

Total Time: 30 minutes

Description: Ignite your dog's senses with this exhilarating beef and broccoli stir fry, abundantly filled with succulent protein and disease-combatting brassicas, igniting vitality and joy!

Ingredients:
1 lb grass-fed sirloin tip, thinly sliced
2 cups broccoli florets
1 medium red bell pepper, julienned
1 medium yellow bell pepper, julienned
1 medium carrot, ribboned or thinly sliced
1 medium onion, quartered and separated
2 cloves garlic, minced
1-inch piece of ginger, grated or finely minced
2 tbsp olive oil or coconut oil
¼ cup low-sodium tamari or coconut aminos
2 tbsp mirin or raw honey
1 tbsp arrowroot powder or cornstarch
¼ cup water or low-sodium organic beef broth
¼ tsp red pepper flakes (optional, for a hint of heat)
Salt and pepper to taste

Instructions:
Commence by preparing all vegetables and meat ahead of time, arranging them close at hand next to the stove.

Blend tamari or coconut aminos, mirin or honey, arrowroot powder or cornstarch, and water or broth in a small bowl, whisking until smooth. Set aside.

Heat oil in a wok or large cast iron skillet over high heat. Carefully place sliced beef into the scalding pan, spreading it out quickly to sear separately in smaller batches. Season with pinches of salt and pepper. Upon achieving beautiful browning, relocate the cooked beef to a separate platter.

In the same invigorating vessel, briefly sauté garlic and ginger merely until releasing their heavenly essence. Interlace the rainbow array of veggies, commencing with harder ones first, namely carrots and onions, followed shortly thereafter by bell peppers and finally broccoli. Distribute saucy mixture evenly over veggies, and constantly agitate to encourage thorough coating.

Crown the splendiferous assembly with previously seared beef, melding it seamlessly back into the ensemble. Allow the symphony to achieve equilibrium for roughly 3-5 minutes, indulging in the spectacle unfolding before you.

Plate with pride, appreciating every colorful element sparking inspiration and anticipation. Savor knows that remnants shall survive refreshingly in the icebox for up to seven days, awaiting future moments of shared pleasure.

Naturally, do recall that corroborating portion dimensions and constituent acceptability with your revered veterinary practitioner or canine nutrition virtuoso serves utmost import, duly acknowledging your admired comrade's singular health preferences and constraints. À table, mes amis!

Dinner Recipes

Pumpkin and peanut butter treats
Yield: Approximately 2 dozen treats

Prep Time: 10 minutes

Cook Time: 20-25 minutes

Total Time: 30-35 minutes

Description: Bestow happiness upon your loyal companion with these delightful pumpkin and peanut butter treats, showcasing nature's bountiful autumn harvest, and delivering wholesome satisfaction!

Ingredients:
2 cups organic whole wheat or gluten-free flour
1 tsp baking powder
1 tsp ground cinnamon
¼ tsp ground ginger
¼ tsp salt
1 cup unsalted creamy peanut butter
1 cup organic canned pumpkin purée (not pie filling)

1 large egg
1 tbsp honey (optional)

Instructions:
First, preheat the oven to 350°F (175°C) and line two cookie sheets with parchment paper or silicone baking mats.

In a medium-sized mixing bowl, whisk together dry ingredients: flour, baking powder, cinnamon, ginger, and salt.

Using a stand mixer or electric beaters, whirl peanut butter, pumpkin purée, egg, and honey (if using) on medium speed until smoothly integrated.

Gradually spoon in the combined dry ingredients, continuing to blend on low speed until the dough forms a firm, cohesive ball.

Turn dough onto a lightly floured surface, kneading gently to eradicate any lingering creases or fractures. Roll out dough to ¼-inch thickness, employing additional flour to deter sticking if need be.

Cut out shapes utilizing favorite cookie cutters, consolidating scraps to repeat the rolling and cutting procedure until all dough has been utilized. Arrange treat rounds neatly on prepared cookie sheets, spacing approximately ½-inch apart.

Deposit tray(s) in the center of the preheated oven, setting a timer for 20-25 minutes, or until visibly crisped and faintly bronzed. Cool completely on wire racks before dispensing liberally unto expectant faces. Remaining treats may be stored in airtight containers for up to ten days, or frozen for extended enjoyment.

Always validate ingredients and measurements with your devoted veterinarian or distinguished canine nutrition sage, staying vigilant towards your noble friend's exceptional health matters and caveats. Joyeux festin!

Carrot and apple training treats
Yield: Around 30 treats

Prep Time: 10 minutes

Cook Time: 20-25 minutes

Total Time: 30-35 minutes

Description: Bolster motivation during teachable moments with these charmingly chewy carrot and apple training treats, celebrating earthy sweetness and fruity tang, rewarding loyalty with love!

Ingredients:
1 cup rolled oats
1 cup organic whole wheat or gluten-free flour
½ tsp baking powder
1 tsp ground cinnamon
¼ tsp ground ginger
¼ tsp salt
1 cup finely grated carrots
1 medium apple, peeled, cored, and grated
1 large egg
2 tbsp melted coconut oil
2 tbsp raw honey

Instructions:
Preheat the oven to 325°F (165°C) and ready two rimmed baking sheets with parchment paper or silicone liners.

In a large mixing bowl, whisk together dry ingredients: rolled oats, flour, baking powder, cinnamon, ginger, and salt.

Make a well amid the dry mixture, introducing wet ingredients: grated carrots, grated apple, egg, melted coconut oil, and honey. Use a spatula to diligently merge the moist and dry components, fashioning a dense, homogeneous batter.

Employing a miniature cookie scoop or rounded measuring teaspoons, distribute dollops of batter onto prepared baking sheets, positioning them roughly 1 inch apart. Flatten tops marginally with fingertips or a fork, ensuring consistent thickness for uniform cooking.

Insert sheets in the middle rack of the preheated oven, programming the timer for 20-25 minutes, or until the peripheries display modest browning. Permit cooling entirely on wire racks before presenting gleefully to eager recipients. Store leftovers in tightly sealed containers for up to two weeks, or freeze them for longer durability.

Never overlook validating recipe details and proportions with your experienced veterinarian or proficient canine nutrition consultant, respecting the individual health inclinations and restrictions of your valued partner.

Note: Always remember to check with your veterinarian or canine nutritionist concerning portion sizes and ingredient suitability based on your dog's specific needs and cancer diagnosis.

Chapter IV. Tips for Transitioning Your Dog to a Home-Cooked Diet

Gradual transition period

Abruptly changing your dog's food may cause gastric distress, loose feces, and other discomforts. Establishing a gradual transition period facilitates a more seamless move towards a home-cooked cancer diet by giving your dog's body time to adjust to new ingredients and textures.

Duration: A good transition should usually take 7 to 10 days. This period should be divided into 25% to 100% increments so that the new diet's proportion may be progressively increased as the old diet's proportion is lowered.

Actions:
Day 1-3: Combine 75% of the prior food with 25% of the new, home-cooked cancer diet.

Day 4-6: Increase to 50% of the new diet and 50% of the previous nourishment.

Day 7–9: Progress to 25% of the traditional cuisine and 75% of the inventive menu.

Day 10: Finally, start feeding all of the freshly implemented, nutritionally complete, home-cooked cancer diet.

Monitoring: Throughout this stage, keep an eye out for any changes in behavior, appetite, waste production, or consistency of the feces. If issues occur, reduce the pace of change briefly and go back to the previous ratio for a few more days before continuing. Always remember that taking care of your dog's delicate stomach pays off in the long run.

Consultation: To confirm the viability and timing of the proposed transition timetable, enlist the assistance of a reputable veterinarian or professional canine nutritionist. Their knowledge is extremely helpful in managing problems caused by pre-existing medical conditions, dietary restrictions, or food allergies. You will plan a smooth transition with the help of your compassionate advisor, supporting your loyal friend in his continuous fight against cancer.

Dog's weight and general well-being

Significance: Consistent monitoring of your dog's weight and general well-being provides valuable information on how well the homemade cancer diet meets their requirements. Small changes in look, demeanor, or physical responses indicate if the recipes chosen provide the best nutrition or need to be adjusted.

Weigh your dog once a week and record the results to see patterns in weight. Aim for consistent, gradual growth or losses following your veterinarian's advice, but be prepared for any slight variations. Extremely unstable readings suggest that changing one's diet would be a good idea.

Body Condition Score: Your veterinarian or an internet scoring table can be used to assess your dog's body composition. Scores typically fall between 1 and 9, which denotes emaciated to severely obese. Aim for a score that falls in the middle, indicating a physically fit and well-balanced body.

Stool Analysis: Every day, pay close attention to your dog's feces and look for any changes in terms of form, color, moisture content, or volume. Logs that are well-formed and light brown indicate good absorption and digestion. Blood, mucus, or diarrhea indicate possible discomfort that needs to be looked at.

Observation of Appetite: Monitor your dog's excitement when it is time for meals, noting any instances of resistance or urgency. Significantly varying interest suggests discontent with the food and may call for changes.

Water Intake Supervision: Keep track of fluid intake patterns and inspect bowls twice a day. Sudden changes indicate underlying issues that need to be investigated.

Documenting Your Dog's Physical Activity: Keep track of your dog's workout regimen, including walks, games, and outdoor adventures. Modifications in your endurance or range of motion notify you of minor health issues.

Frequent Vet Visits: Make appointments with your veterinarian regularly to go over observations, get advice, and get expert opinions. Experts assess global health indicators, respond to inquiries, and suggest modifications, working together to support your attempts to maintain a supporting, well-balanced diet.

In conclusion, keeping a close eye on your dog's weight and general health allows you to make well-informed decisions that will protect their welfare and make the home-cooked cancer diet successful. Using consistent evaluation, dialogue, and adjustment, your cooperation fosters a fruitful alliance committed to battling cancer and promoting enduring health.

Speaking with a dog nutritionist or veterinarian

Professional Advice: Working with a licensed veterinarian or dog nutritionist provides access to knowledgeable individuals who are knowledgeable in complementary cancer therapy, dietary approaches, and customized meal planning. Positive conversations center on goal-oriented assessments, ongoing development, and diagnosis.

Individualization: Each dog facing cancer requires a unique strategy that takes into account their medical history, lifestyle choices, and dietary limitations. Skilled experts evaluate these factors and create aesthetically pleasing, nutrient-dense diets that satisfy specific needs.

Scientific Basis: Well-versed professionals combine scientific literature with real-world applications to create diets based on tested theories and empirical data. Well-informed suggestions conform to established norms, ensuring secure, functional arrangements.

Complementary care: Skilled veterinarians and canine nutritionists realize the significance of integrative care, embracing conventional therapies and alternative techniques. Combinations that work well together can provide significant therapeutic advantages and increase chances for effective cancer treatment.

Ongoing Communication: Positive connections allow for frequent communication, which promotes dynamic evolution in response to changing demands. Continuous cooperation ensures progress and solidifies dedication to high-quality treatment.

Accessibility: Reputable clinics and solo practitioners accept inquiries and provide online consultations, phone conversations, email correspondence, and in-person appointments. Geographical limitations are overcome by virtual platforms, which distribute resources worldwide.

Proactive Measures: Early involvement creates a strong foundation by providing families with pertinent knowledge, resources, and guidelines. Prompt engagement creates the conditions for fruitful conversations, seamless transitions, and satisfying experiences.

Suggested Resources: Look for recognized organizations that support high academic standards, exacting certification requirements, and moral behavior. Prominent organizations are the International Association of Animal Massage and Bodywork (IAAMB) and the American College of Veterinary Nutrition (ACVN).

Reputable vets and dog nutritionists impart priceless knowledge, enabling dedicated people to bravely traverse the world of homemade cancer diets. Optimal health results from professional direction, personalization, a scientific basis, and unceasing engagement interspersed with ongoing education and development. Accept cooperation, opening up countless opportunities for successful cancer adventures.

Conclusion

Embarking on a home-cooked cancer diet marks a transformational step towards promoting canine health and longevity. Acknowledged nutrients, cautiously selected ingredients, and strategic preparations converge, forming a harmonious union of compassion and science.

Understanding canine nutritional needs about cancer illuminates the paramount role of protein, omega-3 fatty acids, antioxidants, and fiber in combating cancer's influence. Likewise, awareness of prohibitive foods averts potential pitfalls, securing progress.

Delicious and straightforward recipes inspire hope, fuelling determination as loving parents endeavor to overcome challenging diagnoses. Meanwhile, gradual transition periods facilitate acceptance, mitigating digestive disturbances.

Meticulous monitoring uncovers nuanced shifts, informing astute decisions aimed at preserving well-being. Ultimately, sought-after improvements emerge, manifesting through radiant eyes, lustrous coats, renewed vitality, and peace of mind.

Collaboration with knowledgeable veterinarians and canine nutritionists ensures expert guidance, individualized solutions, and unwavering dedication. Rooted in mutual trust, fruitful conversations kindle innovation, transformation, and victory.

Together, we forge paths to healing, embracing the power of home-cooked cancer diets and ushering forth a revolution in canine care. Unbounded gratitude resonates, honoring tireless champions of humankind's most loyal allies, forever intertwining hearts, minds, and souls.

First and foremost, congratulations on taking the initial steps toward actively participating in your beloved dog's health journey through proper nutrition! Your unwavering dedication reflects the profound bond you share, and we wholeheartedly celebrate your pursuit of excellence.

Navigating the world of canine cancer care can feel overwhelming, yet armed with curiosity and resolve, countless doors reveal themselves, opening realms of discovery and possibility. The choice to explore home-cooked cancer diets embodies your fierce commitment to nurturing your cherished companion, empowering you both to traverse the road ahead with confidence and grace.

Embraced within these pages lies a wealth of knowledge, inspiring courage, and awakening dreams for a vibrant tomorrow. Cherished memories wait just beyond the horizon, whispering promises of laughter, frolic, and endless adventures. Together, let's harness the magic of holistic nutrition, casting a spellbinding net of hope, healing, and love.

Take heart in the realization that each small stride brings immense rewards, propelling you closer to realizing your ultimate vision. From comprehending the vital roles of essential nutrients to mastering tantalizing recipes, your voyage promises growth, self-discovery, and meaningful connections.

Let us rejoice in the multitudes of victories already achieved, applauding your willingness to invest time, energy, and passion into safeguarding your faithful friend's well-being. And, dear guardians, know that you are not alone. Countless others walk beside you, united in purpose, united in spirit, and united in love.

May the wisdom contained within these words echo through eternity, lighting the way forward, and touching the lives of countless beings blessed to cross your path. Stand tall, radiate kindness, and revel in the magnificent tapestry of existence, unraveled thread by thread, stitch by stitch, breath by breath.

With infinite appreciation and admiration, thank you for entrusting us with the privilege of accompanying you on this incredible adventure. May your spirits soar, your bonds grow, and your love multiply, as you continue to champion the miraculous healing powers inherent in proper nutrition.

All our very best, now and always.

References

ACVIM consensus statement: Nutritional management of dogs and cats with cancer. Journal of Veterinary Internal Medicine, 29(5), 1449–1460. <https://doi.org/10.1111/jvim.14653>

Dodds, J. L., Laverdure, D. R. (2015). *Canine Nutrigenomics: The New Science of Feeding Your Dog for Optimum Health.* DogWise Publishing.

Freeman, L. M., Michel, K. E. (2016). *Clinical evaluation of dietary supplementation for dogs and cats with cancer.* Topics in Companion Animal Medicine, 31(1), 5–11. <https://doi.org/10.1053/j.tcam.2016.01.001>

Henry, C.JK., Murphy, M.J. (2019). *Impact of nutrition on cancer risk and treatment in companion animals.* Journal of Comparative Pathology, 160(2), 107–119. <https://doi.org/10.1016/j.jcpa.2018.11.003>

Lana, S. E., Wood, H. C. (2016). *Natural approaches to cancer in small animals. Veterinary Clinics: Small Animal Practice, 46(5), 981–996.* <https://doi.org/10.1016/j.cvsm.2016.04.005>

MacEwen, E. G., Giles, C., Harvey, H. J., Ogilvie, G. K. (2002). *Results of a prospective study evaluating the effects of dietary modification in dogs with lymphoma receiving multiagent chemotherapy.* Journal of the American Animal Hospital Association, 38(1), 25–31. <https://doi.org/10.5326/15473736-38-1-25>

Rossi, E., Battelli, M., Marcon, F., De Marco, M. L., Brambilla, G., Mosca, F. (2014). *Role of dietary supplementation in patients with spontaneous tumors: Review of clinical trials in dogs and cats.* Journal of Veterinary Pharmacology and Therapeutics, 37(5), 377–390. <https://doi.org/10.1111/jvp.12109>

Shmalberg, J. W. (2016). *Current concepts in nutrition and cancer.* Today's Veterinary Nurse, 7(1), 32–40. <https://www.todaysveterinarynurse.com/current-concepts-nutrition-cancer/>

Watson, A. D., Larson, M. K., Schoenfeld-Tacher, R., Fascetti, A. J. (2017). *Evidence-Based Approaches to Canine and Feline Nutrition.* Elsevier Inc.